VITAMIN K DEFICIENCY

Understanding The Causes, Symptoms, Prevention, Optimal Vitamin K Intake, Recommendations And Considerations

JOSE ASHER

Table of Contents

Introductory

The fat-soluble vitamins known collectively as vitamin K play an essential part in both the clotting of blood and the metabolism of bone.

Because the vitamin is necessary for the production of proteins that are involved in the process of blood clotting, the letter "K" derives from the German word "koagulation." There are two primary types of vitamin K: K1 (phylloquinone), which is found in green leafy vegetables, and K2 (menaquinone), which is created by bacteria in the intestines and is found in fermented foods.

Both types of vitamin K are necessary for proper bone and blood clotting. It is believed that vitamin K contributes to bone health by assisting in the management of calcium levels, in addition to the role it plays in the clotting process. Therefore, it is not only about stopping the bleeding; it is also about maintaining healthy bones!

CHAPTER ONE
Why Vitamin K Is So Important

There are a few primary reasons why vitamin K is important. In the first place, it's necessary for the process by which blood clots. Your body would have a difficult time forming blood clots, which are essential for putting a stop to bleeding after an injury or cut, if you did not get a proper amount of vitamin K.

Vitamin K is important for bone health in addition to its function in the clotting process. Calcium, a crucial element for bone strength, is better regulated as a result of this.

Vitamin K helps to ensure that calcium is deposited in the bones and teeth in the correct manner, which contributes to the bones' and teeth's overall structure and strength.

In addition, evidence suggests that vitamin K may have other health benefits, including as promoting cardiovascular health and lowering the risk of fractures in people who are older.

In conclusion, vitamin K is important since it is a nutrient that serves multiple purposes. It is involved in the process of blood clotting as well as the metabolism of bone, thus making a positive contribution to your general health.

Vitamin K In Its Many Forms

K1 and K2 are the two basic forms of vitamin K that can be found.

• Phylloquinone, a type of vitamin K1 that can be found in green leafy plants including spinach, kale, and broccoli. It is the most common source of vitamin K in the diets of humans and is necessary for the liver's generation of clotting factors.

• Vitamin K2 (Menaquinone): This type of vitamin K2 is produced by bacteria that live in the intestines, and it can also be found in certain fermented foods and animal products. There are 13 different subtypes of vitamin K2, which are designated by the numbers MK-4 to MK-13.

Each subtype is derived from a unique source. It is assumed to serve a role in helping the body control calcium levels and plays a role in the metabolism of bones.

K1 is more related with blood clotting, whereas K2 is more associated with bone health. However, both forms of vitamin K are essential for maintaining overall health.

It's like having two of the most powerful people in the world working together to keep your body under check!

Vitamin K's Many Uses And Functions

Vitamin K is a nutrient that serves multiple critical roles in the body, including but not limited to the following:

• Blood Clotting: The creation of proteins known as clotting factors requires vitamin K, which is essential for this process. These proteins are necessary for the process by which blood clots, which stops excessive bleeding in the case that you have been harmed.

• Bone Health Calcium levels in bones and teeth are regulated in part by vitamin K, which is important for bone health.

It contributes to the synthesis of particular proteins that bind calcium, hence assisting in the development of strong and dense bones.

• The Prevention of Arterial Calcification and Its function in Cardiovascular Health: Some study suggests that vitamin K may play a function in the prevention of arterial calcification and its involvement in cardiovascular health.

This suggests that it may help to maintain the flexibility of your blood vessels and make them less susceptible to hardening.

• Cell Growth and Regulation: Vitamin K is engaged in cellular processes, including cell growth and regulation. One of these roles is cell growth. It is possible that it plays a part in promoting the healthy division of cells.

In general, vitamin K serves a role analogous to that of the stage crew;

it performs its duties in the background to ensure that everything, from blood clotting to bone health, runs well.

It may be a minor nutrient, but it carries a significant burden!

CHAPTER TWO
Sources From The Diet

You may receive the vitamin K you need from a wide variety of foods and drinks in your diet. Some instances are as follows:

1. Vitamin K1 Derived From These Foods:

• Vegetables with Dark Green Leaves: Vitamin K1 can be found in abundance in green leafy vegetables such as spinach, kale, collard greens, broccoli, and Brussels sprouts.

• Oils Extracted from Vegetables: Soybean oil, canola oil, and olive oil all have vitamin K1 in them.

2. Foods Rich in Vitamin K2: Natto, a traditional Japanese dish prepared from fermented soybeans, is one example of a food that is very abundant in vitamin K2.

• Cheese: Gouda and brie are two examples of the varieties of cheese that are high in vitamin K2 content.

• Meat: Some cuts of beef, poultry, and pork, as well as other types of animal products, include trace quantities of vitamin K2 in them.

Keep in mind that the key to ensuring that you consume an adequate quantity of vitamin K is to have a diet that is both balanced and varied. It's a great justification for indulging in a wide variety of mouthwatering dishes!

Maximum Allowable Concentration

It is possible for the amount of vitamin K that should be consumed on a daily basis to differ from person to person depending on age, gender, and existing medical conditions. Nevertheless, the following are some of the general recommendations made by health authorities:

1. For Mature Individuals (both Men and Women):

• The amount of vitamin K1 that should be consumed daily is somewhere between 90 and 120 micrograms on average.

• Vitamin K2: Although there is not a precise suggested daily intake for K2, include sources of K2 in your diet, such as fermented foods, can be beneficial.

2. Vitamin K2 and Children: Vitamin K2 and ChildrenWith increasing age comes a higher RDA (recommended daily consumption). For instance, the recommended dosage for babies is approximately 2 to 2.5 micrograms, but the recommended dosage for teenagers is 75 to 90 micrograms.

These are only some rough recommendations; everyone's requirements are different. It is always a good idea to check with a healthcare professional or a nutritionist in order to identify the appropriate quantity of vitamin K for your individual situation. One another argument in favor of maintaining a healthy equilibrium on your plate!

Causes Of Vitamin K Deficiency And The Symptoms It Produces

A lack of vitamin K can develop for a variety of causes, and when it does, it can cause serious health problems. The following is an explanation of the symptoms and causes:

• Inadequate Dietary Intake: One of the causes of vitamin K deficiency is an inadequate diet, namely one that is lacking in foods high in vitamin K, notably green leafy vegetables and other sources.

• Problems with Malabsorption: Certain medical illnesses, such as celiac disease and cystic fibrosis, as well as problems that affect the bile ducts or pancreas, can interfere with the body's ability to absorb fat-soluble vitamins, including vitamin K.

• The use of antibiotics Certain antibiotics have the potential to upset the natural bacterial balance in the intestines, which can interfere with the creation of vitamin K2 by the bacteria in the intestines.

• Disorders of the Liver Because vitamin K is required for the manufacture of clotting factors in the liver, vitamin K insufficiency can be caused by disorders of the liver.

Signs and symptoms:

• Excessive Bleeding: An increased tendency to bleed is the most common and significant symptom of a deficiency in vitamin K due to the importance of vitamin K in the process of blood clotting.

• Bruising Easily: Because to the impairment in blood clotting, individuals with a deficit may experience bruising easily, even with relatively mild injuries.

• Oozing or Excessive Menstrual Bleeding: Prolonged bleeding from cuts, wounds, or heavy menstrual bleeding in women can be an indication of deficiency. Menstrual bleeding can also be a sign of deficiency.

• Problems with Bone Health Vitamin K insufficiency is uncommon, but it has been linked to lower bone mineral density and an increased risk of fractures.

If you feel that you may have a vitamin K deficiency, it is essential to speak with a medical practitioner in order to receive an accurate diagnosis and appropriate therapy. They could suggest making some modifications to your diet or taking vitamin supplements in order to treat the deficiency and stop any further issues. Don't let those leafy vegetables fall off your plate!

CHAPTER THREE
Advantages To One's Health

Vitamin K has various positive effects on one's health, which demonstrates its significance to one's general wellbeing:

• Blood Clotting Vitamin K is necessary for the manufacture of clotting factors, which is important for ensuring that blood is able to properly clot. This is absolutely necessary for the healing of wounds and stopping of excessive bleeding.

• Contribution to Bone Mineralization and Density Vitamin K is involved in the control of calcium, which is one of the factors that contributes to bone mineralization and density. Having sufficient quantities of vitamin K may assist in the maintenance of strong and healthy bones.

• Contribution to Cardiovascular Health: A number of studies have suggested that vitamin K may play a part in the prevention of arterial calcification. This would contribute to cardiovascular health by ensuring that blood vessels remain flexible.

• Decreased Risk of Fractures Having adequate amounts of vitamin K has been linked to a decreased risk of fractures, particularly in people who are older. It is possible that it will contribute to the strength and integrity of the bones.

• Participation in the Growth and Regulation of Cells: Vitamin K plays a role in the functions of cells, including the growth and regulation of cells. It is possible that it plays a part in promoting the healthy division of cells.

• Possibility of Anti-Inflammatory Effects Vitamin K has been investigated for the possibility that it possesses anti-inflammatory characteristics, which may contribute to an individual's overall health and the prevention of disease.

Consuming foods that are high in vitamin K and including them in your diet can help contribute to the health benefits listed above.

To achieve and sustain general wellbeing, however, it is necessary to keep both one's nutrition and one's lifestyle under check. Therefore, it is imperative that you remember to incorporate those leafy greens and other foods rich in vitamin K into each of your meals.

Interactions With Different Pharmaceuticals

It is imperative that you are informed of any potential drug interactions when taking vitamin K, particularly if you are undergoing a course of therapy that may cause certain side effects. The following are some examples:

• Anticoagulants, also known as blood thinners, are medications that reduce the amount of blood in the body by inhibiting coagulation proteins that are vitamin K dependent.

A rapid shift in one's consumption of vitamin K can have an impact on the efficacy of these medications. Consuming a consistent amount of vitamin K is essential for persons who are on blood-thinning medication.

• Antibiotics: Certain antibiotics, particularly those with a broad spectrum of activity, are known to upset the natural balance of the bacteria that live in the intestines, which in turn interferes with the creation of vitamin K.

• Cholestyramine and Orlistat: These drugs, which are used to decrease cholesterol and help in the process of weight reduction, have the potential to interfere with the absorption of fat-soluble vitamins, including vitamin K.

• Particular Medications for Epilepsy: Vitamin K levels in the body may be lowered by the use of certain medications, such as phenytoin (Dilantin) and phenobarbital.

It is imperative that you keep your healthcare provider updated on any and all dietary changes, as well as any drugs or supplements that you take. They are able to offer direction on how to manage any potential interactions that may occur and ensure that your treatment plan is both safe and effective. Maintaining your health and well-being requires that you keep an open line of contact with your healthcare staff.

CHAPTER FOUR
How To Determine The Appropriate Supplements

When it comes to selecting a vitamin K supplement, there are a few things you should keep in mind to guarantee that you end up with the optimal product, including the following:

• The Variety of Vitamin K Found in Supplements Vitamin K1 or K2 May Be Present in Vitamin K Supplements 1. You might opt to take a supplement that contains the kind of vitamin K that is most appropriate for your objectives, depending on the individual requirements of your health.

• Dosage: The correct dosage can be different for different people depending on criteria such as age, current health status, and particular health issues. It is recommended that you discuss the appropriate dosage for you with your healthcare professional.

• The Supplement Can Be Taken In Many Different Forms In addition to pills and capsules, vitamin K supplements can also be taken in liquid form. Pick a method that fits into your schedule well and is simple to include into your daily activities.

• Quality and Brand: When shopping, look for well-known companies that are committed to maintaining their high level of quality. When purchasing dietary supplements, it is important to be sure that they have been tested and certified by an impartial third party.

• Possible Interactions If you are taking any other medications or supplements, you should talk to your doctor to make sure there won't be any negative side effects from taking the vitamin K supplement at the same time as those medications or supplements.

• Personal Health Goals: Take into consideration the particular health goals you have set for yourself. Regardless of whether you're looking to improve your bone health, cardiovascular function, or overall well-being, selecting a supplement that works in conjunction with your objectives might be useful.

It is important to keep in mind that it is always recommended to consult with your healthcare physician prior to beginning any new supplement regimen. They are able to offer individualized guidance based on your medical history in order to assist you in making well-informed decisions. To compare supplements to sidekicks, you want to be sure you have the correct one by your side!

Conclusion

Vitamin K is a multipurpose nutrient that plays a key role in the maintenance of your health. Vitamin K is a genuine multitasker; in addition to its impact on bone health and possible benefits for the cardiovascular system, it plays a crucial part in the clotting of blood.

The most important things you can do to make sure you get the benefits of this essential vitamin are to include vitamin K-rich foods in your diet, lead a balanced lifestyle, and pay attention to the possibility that certain prescriptions will interact negatively with one another.

Giving vitamin K the attention it deserves, whether it be through the leafy greens on your plate or a supplement that you have carefully selected, helps to the overarching harmony of your health. Allow vitamin K to do its job, which includes assisting your body in clotting blood and strengthening bones, among other things. If you have any questions about vitamin K, your healthcare practitioner is the best person to answer them. They can also help you adjust your strategy to meet the specific requirements of your body. Cheers to living a healthy, well-rounded, vitamin-rich life!

THE END

www.ingramcontent.com/pod-product-compliance
Lightning Source LLC
Chambersburg PA
CBHW060849260726

48661CB00002B/686